101 "Everyday" Secrets for Losing Those Stubborn, Hard To Shed Pounds

By Paul Webb
Olympic Strength & Fat Loss Coach

I0441142

INTRODUCTION

The Good Ol' Days...

It wasn't so very long ago that the need to 'lose weight' or 'burn body fat' was completely unheard of. Indeed, I'll bet that a few short years ago your grandparents would have been mystified by the pursuit of 'six-pack abs!'

People ate heartily and well. This wasn't a concern of course as they worked hard too. They woke up early and engaged in a whole days work, usually doing something that was very physical.

They would work on fields, digging, sowing, harvesting. They tilled the soil, rode horses, worked on farms, ranches etc, and as a result could afford to eat almost anything they wanted, in whatever quantities were deemed necessary.

But that was a long time ago. The world has changed so much in the intervening period. The industrial revolution and development of large modern cities has led to a totally different lifestyle than those of a few generations ago.

We truly are prehistoric man living in the modern world and although we have seen some remarkable advances over the last 50 years, it hasn't always led to the betterment of our health and vitality.

The advent of the internet, for example means we can conduct our lives from the comfort of our living room and, as a result of this, weight gain and ill health has become a major concern for a huge number of the population.

This leads us to an important point. It's not really about the perfectly sculpted, toned physique that adorns the cover of health magazines across the world, it's more about staying fit and remaining healthy to ensure a long, disease free life.

Almost every study on the subject shows that just a few extra pounds of weight over ideal, especially around the stomach, has a huge impact on our health. A switch to a healthier lifestyle not only helps shift those unsightly pounds it also will help to add life to our years.

This tips booket has been written with weight loss (fat loss to be more exact) in mind. This WILL NOT happen by itself. There are different parts of the fat loss jigsaw puzzle that need to be put in place to accomplish our goal...

Firstly by watching what we eat and secondly by taking part in some exercise (sorry, your body needs to move around even if you don't want too) and by also getting a good nights sleep and de-stressing. As you go through the following pages my hope is that you're continually amazed by all the 'everyday' things you can be doing to lose that stubborn body fat!

Let me know how you get on.....

1.

Drink plenty of water. Our body needs a lot of water so give in to it. Water is not just way to flush out toxins but if you have more water in your body you will generally feel healthier and fitter. This itself will discourage any tendency to gorge, especially if you drink some water when you start to feel a little hungry.

The best thing about water is that is has no calories at all.

2.

Start your day with a glass or two of water.

As soon as you wake up, gulp down a glass of cool water. It's a wonderful way to start your day. A glass of water lets out all your digestive juices and sort of lubricates the insides of your body.

It usually means you eat less for breakfast as well.

3.

Drink a glass of water 10 mins before you start a meal. Water naturally needs some space so that you feel fuller without actually having to stuff yourself.

Hunger is also a thirst indicator. By quenching your thirst
before you eat you tend to take on board less calories
than you otherwise would.

4.

Have another glass of water while you are having the
meal. Again this is another way of making yourself full so
that you can actually rise from the table eating less but
feeling full just the same. Instead of drinking it one gulp,
take sips after each morsel. It will help the food to settle
faster so that you get that feeling that you are full faster.

> **SIDENOTE:** Water is such a remarkable thing,
> but seldom do we give it the credit that it
> deserves. Did you know that over 66% of your
> body weight is nothing but water? It's
> amazing!
>
> Water also plays a vital role in weight
> control, which is why I donated so much space
> to it, above.

5.

Stay away from sweetened bottle drinks, especially sodas.

All those colas and fizzy drinks are sweetened with sugar
and sugar means calories. A can of Coke or similar drink
can have the equivalent of 12 to 16 teaspoons of sugar.

The more you can cut back on these sweetened bottle drinks, the better for your fat loss efforts.

Don't think for one minute that sodas are an adequate replacement for water. Remember that we are designed to drink water and water alone, so make the bulk of your fluid intake clean, pure water.

6.

Include in your diet things that contain more water like tomatoes and watermelons. They contain 90 to 95 % water so that there is nothing that you have to lose by feasting on them. They fill you up without adding to the pounds.

7.

Eat fresh fruit instead of drinking fruit juice.

Juice is often sweetened & pasteurised but fresh fruits have natural sugars which the body utilises better than processed sugar. When you eat fruit, you are taking in a lot of fiber, which are needed by the body, and fruits of course are an excellent source of vitamins and other secondary nutrients.

8.

If you do have a craving for fruit juice then go for freshly squeezed instead of those that contain artificial flavours and colours. Or even better, try making your own fruit juice. Just make sure to drink it immediately. The nutrients contained degrade almost straight away.

9.

Choose fresh organic fruit over processed fruits. Processed and canned fruits do not have as much fiber as fresh fruit and are nearly always sweetened.

10.

Increase your fiber intake. Like I mentioned, the body needs a lot of fiber and it plays a huge role in regulating your blood sugar, a vital component of fat loss.

Try to include in your diet as many fruits and vegetables as you can, especially cruciforms vegetables like broccoli, spinach, kale and cauliflower.

11.

Go crazy on vegetables. Vegetables are your best bet when it comes to losing pounds. Always choose vegetables over fruits for maximum weight loss results.

Nature has a terrific spread when it comes to choosing vegetables. And the leafy green vegetables are your best bet. Try to include a salad in you diet always.

12.

Eat intelligently. The difference between man and animal is that we are driven by intelligence while animals are driven by instinct. Don't just eat something because you feel like eating it. Ask yourself whether your body really needs it.

13.

Watch what you eat. Keep a watchful eye on everything that goes in. Sometimes the accompanying garnishes can be richer than the food itself. Remember that it is the easiest thing in the world to eat something without realising that it was something that you should not have eaten. Selective memory you know...

14.

Control that sweet tooth. Remember that sweet things generally mean more calories and a less controlled blood sugar profile.

It is natural that we have cravings for sweet things especially chocolates and other confectionary. Go easy on these things and each time you consume something sweet understand that it is eventually going to add on body fat somewhere.

15.

Fix times to have meals and stick to it.

Try to have food at fixed times of the day. You can stretch these times by half an hour, but anything more than that is going to affect your eating pattern. The result will either be a loss of appetite or that famished feeling which will make you stuff yourself with more than what is required the next time you eat.

16.

Eat only when you are hungry. Some of us have the tendency to eat whenever we see food. We use parties as an excuse to stuff ourselves. Understand that the effect of a whole week of dieting can be wasted by just one day's party food.

Whenever you are offered something to eat do not decline it completely, just break of a nibble so that you appear to mind your manners and at the same time can watch your diet.

17.

Quit snacking in between meals.

Do not fall for snacks in between meals. This is especially true for those who have to travel a lot. They feel that the only time they can get a bite to eat is snacks and junk food.

The main problem with most snacks and junk food is that they are usually less filling and contain a lot of fat and calories. Just think about French fries...tempting but terribly fattening.

18.

Snack on vegetables if you must. You might get the pangs of hunger in between meals. It is something that you can very well control.

Or even better, try munching on carrots. They are an excellent way to satisfy those hungry pangs and are good for your eyes and teeth! Dip them in humous for a great snack.

19.

Go easy on tea and coffee.

Tea and coffee are relatively harmless by themselves. It's when you add the cream and sugar that they become fattening. Did you know that having a cup of tea or coffee that has cream and at least two cubes of sugar is as bad as having a big piece of rich chocolate cake?

20.

Try to stick to black tea/coffee. Black tea or coffee can actually be good for you in moderation. But personally I would like to recommend a non caffeinated tea like red bush or a herbal tea.

We generally take in far too much caffeine than is good for us. This upsets our hormone function leading to a slower metabolism and ultimately more body fat.

21.

Count the calories as you eat. It's a good idea to have an idea of the calories that most food items have. If it is a packed thing then the label is sure to have the calories that the substance has.

22.

Be sure to burn off those extra calories by the end of the week. If you feel that you have consumed more calories than you should have during the week then make sure that you work off those extra calories and keep a strict eye on the diet.

23.

Stay away from fried things. Fried things are an absolute no-no. The more fried things that you avoid, the lesser weight you will gain. Fried things are called so because they are fried in oil or fat. And even if the external oil is drained away, there is still a lot of hidden oil in it so stay away from it.

24.

Do not skip meals. The worst thing you can do while watching you diet is skip a meal. It has just the opposite effect of what you want. You need to have at least four regular meals every day.

25.

Fresh vegetables are better than cooked or canned vegetables. Try to eat your vegetables raw. When you cook them, you are in fact taking away nearly half the vitamins in them. And canned vegetables too are processed and are not nearly half as good as fresh vegetables. When you buy your vegetables it would be a good thing to see if the label says that it is pesticide free. Organic vegetables are the way to go here.

26.

Try not too eat the same foods all the time. Eggs at breakfast are one such example.

Although not inherently that bad continually eating them day after day can cause people to build up an intolerance. In this case it would be best to reduce your intake of eggs to maybe three in a week and then eat other foods at other times.

An intolerance leads to inflammation: inflammation leads to stress: stress leads to fat gain (usually around the stomach!)

27.

Make chocolates a rare luxury and not routine.

Chocolates are not, or at least they should not be a part of your diet. So do not indulge too much in them.

Reach for the organic dark chocolate with at least 75% cocoa in. It may taste more bitter but is much better for you.

28.

Choose a variety of foods from all food groups every day. This is a fine way of keeping deficiency diseases at bay and it helps you to experiment with a variety of dishes and thereby keeping you getting bored of your diet.

29.

If you can say no to alcoholic beverages please do. Alcoholic beverages too are not good for you. Beer can be fattening and the rest of the alcoholic drinks may not be fattening by themselves but after a couple you will be in no position to watch your diet and your appetite too will be something to battle with.

30.

Try to have breakfast within one hour of waking. It's always best to have breakfast within an hour of waking so that your body can charge itself with the energy it needs for the day. The idea is not to wait for yourself to get really hungry.

Breakfast is the most important meal of the day but that does not mean that it should be the most filling meal of the day.

31.

50 to 55% of your diet should be carbohydrates. It is a myth that you should try and avoid carbohydrates when you are on a diet. Carbohydrates are a ready source of energy and so 50 to 55% of your diet should be carbohydrates.

However, depending on amount of weight needed to lose, more of these 50 to 55% should be vegetables, a great source of fibrous carbohydrates.

I would always reach first for the vegetables and secondly for low glycemic carbohydrates like sweet potatoes, yams and brown rice.

32.

25 to 30% of your diet, at least, should be proteins.

Various processes and activities are going on in our bodies. Things are broken down and being built up again. Resistance has to be built up, recovery from disease too is needed and for all this the body needs plenty of proteins so see to it that 25 to 30 % of your diet consists of proteins.

I would also add that if your activity level is high, look to consume more high class proteins.

33.

Fats should only be 15 to 20 %. You need only this much of fat in your diet so keep it at that.

Bear in mind though that fat has to be consumed using quality, unaltered fats such as those found naturally in nature. Fat is highly reactive and as such will turn toxic under heat. If cooking with fats please use more stable fats such as butter or coconut fat.

Trying to take all fat out of your diet is not only impossible it's not recommended.

34.

Try and adopt an almost vegetarian diet.

An almost vegetarian diet can be better for those of us watching our diet. There are a lot of advantages of keeping to a vegetarian diet but I don't want to sing an ode to vegetarianism now. What I would suggest is keep to a vegetarian diet as much as you can. I'm often amazed at how few vegetables people eat these days.

Just be careful not to overeat carbohydrates.

35.

Choose white meat rather than red. White meat, which includes fish and fowl, can be better than red meat, which includes beef and pork, for those trying to lose weight.

Go for high class, free range, organic meat as much as possible.

36.

High Fiber multigrain breads are better than white breads. Remember how I told you to increase the fiber content in your food; well this is an answer to that. It is not only better in terms of the fiber content but also in terms of the protein content as well.

WARNING: Be careful if wheat is a problem for you though. Remember we spoke of intolerances to foods earlier. A huge amount of people are wheat intolerant and if this is the case it is probably better to leave the breads alone.

37.

Reduce your intake of pork. Research indicates that pork is not something that can help you to lose weight. So the lesser pork you eat the better chances you have of losing weight. And remember that pork includes the pork products as well, things like bacon, ham and sausages.

38.

Limit your sugar intake. **This is very important!** If you can't have things unsweetened try to use stevia. This is a natural herb that will sweeten with no fat gaining potential.

Don't reach for the sweeteners instead. Research has shown time and time again that they increase body fat and are known to contribute to other health problems.

39.

Graze 4 to 5 times a day. Instead of sticking to just three meals a day, try grazing. Grazing means try having 4 or 5 smaller meals instead of three king sized meals. It is an excellent way of having smaller quantities of food.

40.

Go ahead and treat yourself from time to time. There are many things which you have to avoid from your diet but which you may have an undying craving for. Do not avoid them altogether. You could call them cheat foods and indulge in them once in a while.

But take care just to make it a cheat meal, NOT a cheat day.

41.

Watch your total fat intake. Each fat gram contains 9 calories so by reading the total calories on a food and knowing the quantity of fat, you can estimate the % of fat, which should in no way exceed 30% of the food.

42.

Go easy on salt, as too much salt is one of the causes of obesity. Make it a point to really cut down on your salt intake as much as possible. A small pinch of clean natural sea salt is permissible.

43.

Change from salted butter to salt free free butter. It is healthier for you and tastes just the same. Bear in mind that these small changes can go a long way towards weight reduction.

44.

Instead of frying things try baking them without fat. Baking is by far a healthier method of preparing food than frying. Baking requires lesser oil or fat.

45.

Use a non stick frying pan for your cooking so that you do not have to add oil. The golden rule is to try and avoid as much oil as possible and a non stick pan is the perfect solution to this problem.

46.

Boil your vegetables instead of cooking them, or even better, eat them fresh and raw. However if you do not like eating your vegetables as it is, try steaming them without adding anything at all. This is probably the

healthiest way to eat cabbages, cauliflowers and a host of
other vegetables.

47.

Carry parsley with you. Parsley is an excellent thing to
munch on in between meals. Not just is it good for you in
terms of vitamins, but it is also a perfect way of making
your breath fresher.

48.

Shop wisely. There are plenty of different foods available
in the market so why not choose from a wide range
instead of the same few foods over and over again. Many
people just go for shopping and pick up out of habit.
In the markets of today, you will be astounded at the
range of goods that manufactures have to offer.
Remember that our bodies need nutrients and not just
calories. A wide range of foods will give us all the
nutrients we need.

49.

Avoid crash diets. They are bad for your overall health
and you won't be able to keep the weight off. Crash diets
are not a solution to weight loss. It might seem as if you

have lost few pounds but the moment you give up on the crash diet every thing will bounce back with a vengeance.

Take a look at it in this way. Do you think that it is possible for a person to survive on a crash diet for the rest of his or her life? Certainly not! So at some time or the other, you will have to give up the crash diet and then you will see for yourself that a crash diet does more harm than good on the long run.

Crash diets may have a lot to promise, but very rarely do these promises ring true. Crash diets are things people go on in order to wear an old dress or suit for a particular occasion. That's the only purpose that they serve as far as I can see.

50.

Nature gave us teeth for a reason...

Therefore we should develop a habit of chewing all food including liquid food and soft foods as much as possible. This is essential to add saliva to the food, as it is only in the saliva that sugar is digested.

Often we find that whatever goes into our mouth goes down like lightning. We hardly give the saliva any time to act on the food. So does digestion take place like it should? Do we just stuff our tummies with food that doesn't get digested or in other words that doesn't yield the benefits that it should?

51.

If you choose to drink wine dry is better than sweet.

Sweet wines naturally contain a lot of sugar. But on the other hand, in dry wines most of this sugar has been fermented away so from the weight point of view dry wines are better than sweet wines.

52.

When you decide it's time to start working out, start slowly and don't get discouraged if you don't achieve your fitness goals after the first week. Many people make this mistake. They feel that if they really push their bodies they can lose more weight in a couple of work outs.

If you try to push your body too much initially, you are likely to end up with sprained joints, a sore back and even torn ligaments. The rule to be followed here is slow and steady wins the race.

53.

Check your weight before you start the routine and keep checking for changes but do not expect a radical change immediately, it might be one or two weeks before you notice some change. However it is crucial that you continue to monitor your weight. You may bear in mind the fact that even a few pounds loss is a big achievement.

54.

When you do notice a change, reward yourself. When I say reward I do not mean go for some goodies like chocolates or sweets. Maybe you could go for a movie or buy yourself something.

This is something that can keep you going. It is a good idea to save the money that you wanted to spend on ice creams and chocolates and then treat your self to something more substantial.

55.

You can take a day off from exercise every week. This is not just a very good idea but it is part of the exercise routine. Your body needs a day off from an exercise routine so do not hesitate to take a day off from what ever you have been doing.

56.

Exercise outside as often as possible. There are two advantages of doing whatever you are doing outside. One advantage is that it gives your body a chance to get a lot of the much needed fresh air and sunshine.

The second advantage is that the surroundings keep you perked up and it is a break form remaining cooped up all day long

57.

Try to collect some information about exercise. There are a lot of things that you can do at home. Extensive research has been done on exercise and plenty of this information is easily available.

You can try incorporating the use of an exercise professional, browsing the net, or getting a book or two on how to exercise at home.

This information will be useful to you to know how much you need to work out on each specific exercise in order to burn off the desired number of calories.

58.

Try to get somebody to exercise along with you. But it should be somebody committed or else your interest might dwindle. This is an excellent idea. One of the advantages of getting a committed person to exercise with you is that it keeps you going.

There may be days when you feel just too lazy to crawl out of bed in the mornings. On such days, the knowledge that somebody is waiting for you is enough to slide out of bed.

Another advantage is that you can discuss your progress and fears with another person and be a sympathetic listener to the other person as well. This is a fine way of getting motivated your self.

I often think this is one of the most important things you can do to help with your fat loss. Having a strong support group around you is vital to keep you going.

59.

Stop when your body has had enough. There is no sense in pushing it. When you have worked out enough, your body will start giving you signals.

Heed those signals. This is particularly true in the initial stages. Take one step at a time. Stop when you are out of breath or when a certain part of your body tells you that it has had enough.

60.

If you want to increase your time of exercise or your work out routine, do it gradually and not in sudden steps.

Well easier said than done. Most of us have such hectic schedules that it is quite impossible to fit in tie for exercise right? Wrong. I want to say it once and for all, your body, or anyone's body for that matter needs proper exercise. If you make up your mind to do it, you absolutely can.

61.

Select an exercise pattern to suit your life style. All of us have different life styles and professions so there is no sense in trying to follow the book strictly.

Try and follow an exercise routine that is suitable for you. You have to understand that even more important than the exercise itself is sticking to it. So unless you choose something that can suit your life style, you are not going to be consistent enough to benefit.

62.

Don't stand, walk. If you can walk about then do so. Do not stand in a fixed position. Pacing about is a good thing to do. If you are thinking deeply about something, try pacing about, it will aid in your thinking.

63.

Don't sit, stand. If you can stand, then do not sit. The golden rule is to choose a position that is less comfortable.

64.

Don't lie down, sit. The rule that we mentioned above rings true here as well.

65.

Try not be a sedentary. It is the easiest thing in the world to become a couch potato. You know what we are talking about don't you? That shapeless thing that sits or reclines on a shapeless chair in front of the television and steadily munches away on something fried!

If you are inclined to become a promising old couch potato, break the habit, cut at the very root of the vine. And you want to know what is the best way for that? Take away that favourite chair of yours. In fact, it would be a very good idea if you could keep a chair that isn't too comfortable in front of the TV!

This will discourage any tendency to become a couch potato.

66.

If you have a sitting job, stand up and stretch yourself every hour. Most of the jobs today are indeed sitting jobs that are in very sedentary. This is especially true for those who sit and punch away at the keyboard or toy with the mouse all day long.

So if you have such a job, make it a point to get up at least every half an hour and stretch your self. You could combine this with drinking a glass of clean pure water.

67.

While making telephone calls try walking up and down. I hope you will agree with me that this is an excellent suggestion.

I know of clients who have tried this with great success as they had a habit of sitting on the phone and absent mindedly snacking on biscuits or other fatty snacks.

68.

Use the stairs instead of the elevator whenever you can. Elevators are fantastic, particularly if you have to go up or down some twenty floors. But they also make us very lazy.

There may be no sense in trudging up some twenty flights of stairs because by the time you get there you will be totally pooped. But while coming down, if you have the time, you can easily come down the stairs instead of using the elevator. Coming down is not at all exhausting.

And certainly head for the stairs if you only have a few floors to go up.

69.

Quit smoking. Smoking as such may not contribute to weight loss but smoking leads to other conditions like erratic eating habits and excessive dependence on things like coffee.

It will also leave you particularly breathless when trying to exercise. This will have a big impact as to how much body fat you can burn through exercising.

70.

If you hate running, **good news!!** You do not have to run a marathon each day to stay fit and burn body fat. In fact recent research shows it may actually inhibit your ability to do so.

Instead, work in short sharp bursts with minimal rest periods. 10-20 minutes each day, depending on how hard you work, is good enough for most.

71.

What if you're not fit enough for that? Then start with walking.

15 minutes of brisk walking a day is enough to keep most fit, and when you can move to no.70.

72.

Any distance is walkable, if you have the time. So consider walking to places that you would normally drive (such as work or the market if they're not too far away). It may take you longer, but the health benefits will last you a lifetime.

73.

It sounds strange, but some scientists have reported that people can lose more weight when they drink green tea before a workout.

While there's no hard data to support this, nutritionists speculate that the caffeine in green tea makes the body rely more on fat for fuel during the work out. It's worth trying!

74.

Here's the caveat to the tip above: Avoid drinking green tea in excess, as it tends to desensitize your body to the fat burning effects of caffeine!

No one said this would be easy!!

75.

Stop using remote controls. Remote controls are the bane of a prospective weight loser. They may be remarkable gadgets by themselves but from the weight loss point of view, they just aren't very helpful.

They really encourage us to take a laid back kind of attitude towards life itself. In fact if remote controls were not there, the television would not have become so popular. It is because of remote controls that people can remain where they are and switch from one channel to the other. And they only have to twitch a finger muscle to achieve this.

Now, I have nothing against multi channel television sets but what I strongly advocate is that you get up from where you are and change the channel of the TV each time you want to do so.

The same thing holds true for other remote controls as well. As it is we have remote controlled TVs, DVD players, A/Cs, garage doors, gateways and what not. The next thing we know is that we will have remote controlled people as well.

76.

Do things like fetching, turning things off and on by yourself. Often when we come back tired from work, we tend to get others to do simple chores for us. These things are no big deal. They are things that we can very well do for ourselves but we don't.

That is why we often ask our kids to fetch us this or take away that.

Training your pet is a wonderful thing indeed. It is quite remarkable how some people get their dogs to fetch them something. But the fact is that while you may be making sure that your dog is getting a lot of exercise, you are neglecting your bit of the story.

77.

Here's a pop quiz. Escalators help us to:

1. Move up and down faster
2. Gain weight
3. Stand stupidly as they move up and down
4. Look down at other people when you are going down
5. Look up to others when we are going up

You have to pick the correct answer from the 5 alternatives given. You can see for your self that all the options are in a way correct. So the next time you travel on an escalator, don't just stand there...climb up or down along with it. (Or better yet, take the stairs.)

78.

During commercial breaks walk about or drop and perform a couple of push ups.

When the next commercial flashes on screen, instead of surfing, get up and do something. Reach over and try to touch your toes or do any such simple exercise that will at least get the blood flowing in your veins. Make it a competition with yourself to see how many pushups you can do while the commercials are on.

79.

Wriggle your toes and your fingers whenever you can. This is a stress buster and it gives you a chance to at least work your hand and leg joints. This will tell you how sore they are and if their condition is so bad, just think of the rest of your body.

80.

Turn on music and just dance. Let your hair down once in a while. Go back to the days of your childhood. Close the door of your room, turn on your sound system to the highest volume possible (but a little lower than the level at which your neighbours start to complain) and then do the wackiest dance that you can think of. Jump on your bed and jump off it again.

Roll all over the floor. Pretend that you are Michael Jackson or Madonna (you will never see them keeping still) and do every move that you know.

Just follow the lead of your children.

81.

Carry a soft flying disc or Frisbee with you on your jog or walk. Toss it around and get up to fetch it. This is also an excellent way to beat stress. It makes a person feel good to throw something away forcefully when the person is all worked up. And the thing that you throw is something soft and can't damage anything, then what is stopping you?

It is not really the throwing part that we are interested in. It is the fetching part. Each time you get up to fetch it back; you are giving yourself a chance to stretch those muscles and joints

82.

Get off the tube a stop early and walk the rest of the way. You might not have time to fit in long walks in your busy schedule so this is one way of ensuring that you at least get to perform some card during your day.

If you drive to work, see if you can get space in a parking lot that is a little away from your office.

83.

When nobody is watching try doing pelvic gyrations. If you take a moment to observe it you will see that it is the mid section of our body that gets the least bit of exercise and that is probably why the signs of weight gain are mostly seen there.

It is the same reason why we find it very difficult to lose weight in that section. So the best thing that you can do is consciously try to give that part a little bit of exercise.

Stomach crunches might be too strenuous an exercise to start off, and not suited to a lot of people, but gyrations are relatively mild. Pelvic gyrations make you thrust your midsection towards all directions and this is the best way of tightening every muscle in that mid section and that is of course what weight loss is all about.

These are especially beneficial if done sitting on top of a stability ball. The instability of the ball increases the work rate of your deep abdominal muscles and the more muscular activation the better.

84.

Tuck in your tummy whenever you walk. Get that proper posture. And the best way for that is to tuck in your tummy and inflate your chest. Do not let your tummy hang above your belt line like some unruly layer of flesh. Bring it under the belt.

Each time you tuck in your tummy, you will feel the pressure on the muscles of your stomach. This tightening and loosening of these muscles is even better than stomach crunches.

85.

Try breathing exercises. You might be surprised to know that breathing exercises too can lead to weight loss. If you are doing the breathing exercises properly, you will find that you can exert a lot of pressure on the muscles around the mid section.

You can feel a tightening of these muscles each time you breathe in or breathe out. So go ahead and breathe properly, it is good for you. Just make sure your in breath is deep into the diaphragm and not high in the chest.

86.

Try yoga. Yoga is one of the best ways of losing weight.

One of the benefits of yoga is that you learn to control virtually every muscle and joint of your body so that your flexibility and mobility will increase. This means your range of movement will increase so you are able to increase muscle activation and ultimately burn more body fat.

87.

Try massage.

This is something you can get down with a good therapist or with your partner.

In fact it is a good idea if couples take up weight loss routines together. They can keep watch over each other, help control those urges to eat and motivate each other to stick to the programme .

Massage increases blood flow, soothes sore muscles and just helps the body to function that little bit better.

88.

If you can't think of any thing else to do try punching your pillow. Now here's another one of those weird ideas but believe me it works. Not too many of us have punch bags at home but if you have a really fluffy pillow you could certainly work up a sweat pretending to be Rocky Balboa.

This is also a nice way of letting off steam so go for it. After all something is better than nothing. But I would suggest that you do not hit it too violently or else the stuffing might come out. Do not bother too much about the force with which you hit the pillow. It is number of hits that are important. Try to get at least fifty punches in one bout.

89.

Instead of walking up and down the staircase one at a time, try taking them two or even three at a time.

Now this is something that you have to be careful about so make sure that your feet are well and truly planted on each step before you increase the height of your steps.

90.

If you have a dog, take it for a run and let the dog lead you on. You will be surprised as to how much exercise a dog can give you.

Animals are sensible enough to know that they need a lot of exercise so let your animal lead you on. Take your pet dog out for as walk and before you know what hit you, it will turn out to be a run.

91.

Join a dance class. Dancing is a wonderful way to burn off those extra calories. It is true. When you dance you are in fact burning away a lot of calories. Of course we are not referring to the slow ballroom kind of dances in which one person actually leans on the other one for support. We are talking about fast dances.

The best way to do it is by joining a dance class because they will really wok you out and help a lot with technique.

92.

Whenever you can, lean against a wall with your hands flattened against the wall and in such a way that your face is very close to the wall. Then use you hands to push your body away from the wall. Do this two or three times at a stretch.

You could also sit up and down on your office chair.

In fact challenge yourself to make your work environment a mini gym and see how many exercises you can create with what is around you.

93.

If there is a pool nearby go for a swim as often as you can.

Swimming is a fantastic form of exercise, and if nothing else, a cool dip in a pool is a wonderful stress reliever.

94.

Try playing something like table tennis or badminton.

Games are a fun way to lose weight. It is much more exciting to play a game than just work out by yourself. The best thing about games is that they are addictive. Once you start playing you will soon end up with a friends' circle and then the playing goes on without even you knowing it.

It is something that you can look forward to and there is no stress involved in this programme. In fact the more you play the less you will consider this to be a part of

your weight loss program. As you burn away those
calories, you will also be able to expand your social circle.

95.

Any work out should start with a 5 to 10 minute warm up
and should end with a 5 to ten minute cool down session.
Whatever physical exercise you are involved in, you must
remember to warm up before the exercise really starts.
Do not just plunge into the water and start thrashing
about, to put it figuratively.

Your body needs to reach a certain level of readiness
before it can actually start responding to exercise. And
this readiness is achieved by the warming up process.

96.

Do not carry your mobile phone around but leave it a
place where you can hear it ringing. In this way you make
sure that you at least get up and walk towards it. This
might sound sill but I really mean it. You need a reason to
keep yourself going.

Life today has become so easy that we have every thing
at our fingertips. All we have to do is push a button here
and push a button there. The only things that get any
exercise at all are our fingers. Years ago Charles Darwin
put forward a theory of use and disuse.

According to this theory, a certain part of the body that is put to constant use develops a lot and a certain part of the body that has no use at all becomes smaller and smaller and gradually ceases to exist.

Certain examples that he quoted were the long neck of the giraffe, which appeared to become longer and longer when the giraffe stretched higher and higher to reach the leaves at the treetops. He quoted the example of the absence of a tail in human beings to illustrate the example of the theory of disuse.

Now if Darwin's theory were to prove true, as the years go by man is likely to end up with just a huge head, a few fingers and maybe some other parts of the body that are also put to use.

That is why I made it a point to say that you have to drive your self to move about. A mobile phone may be convenient, but the same thing can turn out to simplify life just a little too bit. There are other arguments against the use of mobile phones but that is not our topic today.

What I would suggest is that at home or in your office, leave the mobile phone lying about so that you can hear it ring, but can't just reach into your pocket and answer it. See to it that you have to actually stand up and walk a few steps before you can pick it up.

97.

While traveling in an elevator instead of just standing there and staring stupidly at the numbers going up or down, try raising your self onto your toes and then back on your feet again. Do this several times. Also try flexing your buttock muscles as well.

In fact there are many muscles in our body that we can twitch and flex without inviting the attention of others. Even if others do notice you, its no big deal provided you are flexing a muscle in a decent part of the body. (Most of the other parts do not have muscles any way.) Others might brand you as a health freak but it is miles better to be known as a health freak than as a sack of potatoes.

98.

Undress and stare at yourself in front of your mirror. If what you see displeases you, then you have all the more reason to work out. Try tucking in the extra fat in all those wide areas, this will give you an idea of which part you need to be working on.

Turn to you side and get a very good view of your side profile. This is an excellent way of checking whether you have a tummy that is starting to bulge or has bulged already.

Try pulling in air and then take a look at your tummy, if it has gone in even a little bit, there is hope for you. If you start now, you can control it where it is now and may be if you really set your mind to it, you can lose a couple of inches in a just a few weeks.

Weighing your self on your bathroom scales is a good idea but personally I would recommend this mirror viewing. To be very frank, a few pounds gain may shock you but does not really disgust you. But a flabby figure and extra fat certainly will.

99.

If you have a banister rail or a balustrade that will support you, sit on it and pump your legs as if you are riding a bicycle, taking care not to fall off of course.

This might sound like another crazy idea and I don't want to argue with you about that. I just want to tell you that by doing such crazy things, you are in fact not missing a single chance to lose those extra pounds. It is a way of keeping your mind alert all the time. Every thing must look like an opportunity to you.

100.

Do not slouch in your chair but try to maintain an erect posture with your tummy tucked in. Slouching is a very bad habit. Not only is it bad for your back but it also gives you a very flabby figure. It is your way of saying yes to a comfortable, weight-gaining pose.

Make it a point to always sit as erect as you can. It is also a terrific way to ward off back problems.

101.

Psst. I would like to let you in on a secret. As it is I understand that most of us tend to put on weight particularly in the mid section, right. It is the tummy that seems to have a mind of its own. Well I will tell you a sure shot method to reduce the flab around the waist line. Mind you this doesn't hold true for post pregnancy tummies. This is what you have to do.

Breathe in air as strongly as you can and as you do so, tuck in your tummy as much as you can. Hold it like this for a few seconds and then slowly release your breath taking care not to let out your tummy. Try to keep breathing like this at least fifty or sixty times in a day.

In fact breathe like this whenever you can remember to do so. After the first day, you should feel the muscles of your stomach tightening each time you do this. Then you know that you are on the right track. If you practice this without fail for 20 days, at the end of the twentieth day, you will have lost at least an inch.

Below I have included a table of the various exercises and the number of calories that can be burnt with each exercise. Choose what you can do best and choose something that you will enjoy doing on the long run as well.

The choice of the exercise is completely left to you but try to do whatever you wish to do for at least twenty minutes. It is only after you do the exercise for twenty minutes that the actual calorie burning sets in.

Aerobics
200-250 calories
Bicycling, Stationary
250-300 calories
Bicycling, Actual
300-400 calories
Running, 5-6 mph
300-350 calories
Stair climber
200-250 calories
Swimming laps
350 calories
Walking briskly
150-180 calories

From this you can see for yourself that walking is not at all something that has to be sidelined. If you really find your days to be too full to fit in any other form of exercise, then walking is your best bet. Walk as much as you can.

Try getting to places and leaving places a little early. This will give you time to walk.

Well, I guess that's about it. The ball is now in your court so what are you waiting for? Get rid of those extra calories and pounds as early as you can and try to enjoy life the best you can without inviting all those terrible diseases that come with a few extra pounds.

About the Author.

Paul Webb is a former professional footballer whose career was cut short by injury. He is the founder of Complete Coaching Ltd, a health and fitness company based in Wanstead, East London, England.

Dissatisfied with the level of care the usual gymnasium offers its members, Paul and his wife Liza decided to set up their own gym making client results and the experience they receive their priorities.

Paul has vast experience in the health and fitness industry having trained and worked with leading coaches here in the UK and overseas in the US.

Working out of the Complete Studio, Paul specialises in coaching clients toward their health and fitness goals and getting athletes stronger and more explosive.

Paul works closely with the Tessa Sanderson Academy and Foundation, offering strength coaching to current and future British athletes. He has also just been appointed head of strength and conditioning for the elite GB Ice Skating Squad.

Paul is married with 4 children.